The Gift of Hope

The Path to Healing through Upper Cervical Chiropractic

Dr. Larry Arbeitman, DC
Dr. George Gertner, DC

Disclaimer

The information in this book is intended for educational use only and should not be construed as medical advice. You should consult with your physician before attempting any activity or making any lifestyle changes discussed in this book. Although every attempt is made to ensure the accuracy of the information presented, the author and publisher are not liable for any illness or injury that may result from attempting any activities or lifestyle changes presented in this book.

Center Path Publishing
14859 Embry Path
Apple Valley, MN 55124

The paper used in this publication meets the minimum requirements of the American National Standards for Information Services - Permanence of Paper for Printed Library Materials, ANSI Z39.48-1984.

We would like to dedicate this book to the thousands of people throughout the years who have trusted us with their health. Thank you for your confidence.

Table Of Contents

1 • Health Is Not Just the Absence of Disease   1

2 • How Your Body Works   5

3 • An Introduction to Chiropractic   37

4 • NUCCA Chiropractic   59

5 • Our Patients Speak   67

1

Health Is Not Just the Absence of Disease

Pain is an important signal that the body is having trouble, and it needs to be taken seriously. It is much like a warning light in the dashboard of your car. Most people would immediately take their car in to be repaired if a warning light appeared in their dashboard. They know that if the problem is not corrected, their car will break down. When the body's warning light comes on—you experience pain—too often, people just ignore it or cover it up with medication. Taking pain-relieving medication only serves to mask your body's "warning light;" it does not actually fix the problem, it only covers it up. It is like putting a piece of black tape over the warning light in your car so you don't have to look at it. You don't feel any pain, but your body continues to break down.

Health is Not Just the Absence of Disease

Health is not just the absence of disease any more than wealth is an absence of poverty. Simply 'feeling fine' does not mean you are healthy, for we know that many serious health problems may progress for years without causing any symptoms. Hypertension and diabetes are perfect examples. They may progress unnoticed for years, and by the time they are discovered, the outcome is often grim.

On the other hand, it is also very common for people to suffer from chronic, low-grade inflammatory or allergic conditions, and be told that there is nothing wrong with them. This is especially true when it comes to poorly understood conditions such as fibromyalgia, chronic fatigue syndrome, chemical sensitivities, and the like. Far too many people are told that their problem is either "in their head" or that it is "nothing to worry about." Even more dangerous is when people simply try to mask the symptoms of their physical problems by covering them up with drugs, such as ibuprofen, antacids, decongestants, and analgesic creams.

Unfortunately, much of the United States health care system is geared towards managing pain and symptoms, rather than working to eliminate the cause of the pain. Going to your family medical doctor usually results in coming home with a prescription for medication that often does nothing to correct the actual problem. This has lead to the American population being overmedicated and unhealthy. There are certainly times when traditional medicine can do amazing things, especially in treating trauma and infectious disease. However, we are currently in the midst of an epidemic of degenerative diseases that traditional medicine is ill-suited to deal with. It is an ineffective and extraordinarily expensive means of disease management.

Upper Cervical Chiropractic: A Healthier Choice

With all of the choices in health care, it is sometimes hard for the average person to know what to do. The constant bombardment with drug advertisements that promote the idea that a pill is the answer to all your health concerns, the limitations on health care access imposed by health management organizations, the endless stream of new "wonder supplements" that claim to cure everything from bad breath to cancer, coupled with the well-intentioned advice of family and friends, has left most people unsure of what to believe.

Unfortunately, one of the most effective means of treatment for a wide variety of conditions from back pain, to headaches, allergies, dizziness, high blood pressure, and problems with digestion is rarely discussed. This treatment is called Upper Cervical Chiropractic.

In this book, you will learn a different way of thinking about your body: one that focuses on the concept that most "disease" states are caused by some form of interference with the body's ability to regulate itself, and that the most important regulatory organ in the body is the central nervous system—comprised of the brain and spinal cord. As you will see, the goal of care is to identify and remove the source of the interference, thereby allowing the body to heal naturally and maintain its own vitality without the need for drugs or surgery.

2

How Your Body Works

There were two things that I vividly remember from an embryology class I took while in chiropractic school. The first was the incredible complexity and mystical wonder of the development of the human body, and the second was understanding why the nervous system is so critical to normal development and health. Starting at conception, the body begins to take shape, beginning with the development of a long cylindrical tube that forms the spinal cord. From this cord, little bumps begin to form that make up all of the internal organs as well as the arms and legs. This process continues, seemingly by magic, for nine months until a fully formed human being emerges. As long as all of the organs function in a tightly controlled balance, the child will continue to thrive and grow into a healthy adult.

While you sit calmly reading this, your body is bristling with activity. The trillions of cells that make up your body are busy at work performing thousands of delicately balanced processes that make your life possible. The brilliance with which your body controls this profoundly complex dance of chemistry is truly divine. And as long as your body is able to keep the dance going, you remain healthy and vibrant. But if there is a disruption in any of the body's processes, the entire system loses its ability to perform correctly and disease emerges.

The body's ability to regulate and control the delicate balance of all of the necessary life processes is called "homeostasis." The term homeostasis is derived from the Greek words for "same" and "steady." It refers to way the body acts to maintain a stable internal balance. For example, your body works to maintain a carefully regulated internal temperature of 98.6 degrees. If you go outside on a warm day and begin to work, your body will begin to sweat in an effort to keep your temperature from increasing too far. You may also begin to breathe deeper in an effort to keep your tissues supplied with oxygen during a period of increased demand.

Disease and disability result whenever the body is stressed beyond its ability to maintain homeostasis. This stress can come in three forms, physical, chemical, and emotional, and always manifests from lifestyle choices such as poor diet, lack of exercise, and excessive emotional stress. Stress always affects the nervous system, resulting in interference or irritation of the nervous system which is the master controller of the body. In this chapter, you will learn about the systems in your body that are necessary for maintaining health. We will briefly talk about the digestive system, cardiovascular system, and immune system, and follow that up with a much more in-depth discussion of the largest system of your body, the neuromusculoskeletal system – your nerves, muscles, and bones.

Digestive System

When we eat such things as bread, meat, and vegetables, they are not in a form that the body can use. Everything that we eat and drink must be broken down into smaller molecules before they can be absorbed and used by the body. This process is called digestion.

The digestive system includes the digestive tract and its accessory organs, which process food into molecules that can be absorbed and utilized by the cells of the body. Food is broken down, bit by bit, until the molecules are small enough to be absorbed and the waste products are eliminated. The digestive tract, also called the alimentary canal or gastrointestinal (GI) tract, includes the mouth, esophagus, stomach, small intestine, and large intestine.

As long as this system works correctly, the nutrients you consume are able to be extracted and absorbed into the bloodstream to be delivered to your individual cells. The digestive system is the means by which you get all of the individual nutrients that are needed for health. Every single molecule in your entire body arrived there in the same way—at some point in the recent past you ate it. This is an important concept to remember because if your diet does not include everything that your body needs, you will lose some of the richness of your health. Consuming food is much like depositing money into your checking account. If you don't have enough resources there, you can't afford to keep fixing your house.

One aspect of digestion that is often overlooked is the role of the nervous system. The mind-body connection between the central nervous system and the digestive system has been well established by science. Most people have heard that stress can lead to gastric ulcers, gastric reflux, and indigestion, as well as diarrhea and constipation. But most people are surprised to discover that the nervous system can also affect food allergies, how nutrients are utilized by the body, and even affects what nutrients the body requires. For these reasons, any time that there is any problem with the digestive system, it is important to consider neurological influences as part of a thorough evaluation.

Cardiovascular System

The cardiovascular system is sometimes called the circulatory system, and consists of the heart, which is a muscular pumping device, and a closed system of vessels called arteries, veins, and capillaries. The role of the cardiovascular system in maintaining homeostasis is the transportation of nutrients and oxygen from the digestive system to all of the cells in the body, as well as the transportation of waste and carbon dioxide to be eliminated.

As long as your cardiovascular system works correctly, your body has an enormous capacity to adapt to just about any external demand. For example, when you begin to exercise, your heart pumps faster and your blood pressure increases in order to supply more oxygen and nutrients to your tissues. When you are cold, your blood vessels constrict in some areas of the body—the back of your arm, for instance—in an effort to conserve heat. When your body is injured, the blood vessels open up to allow white blood cells to enter the area to fight infection and speed healing.

Unfortunately, the cardiovascular system is the one that fails most often due to an unhealthy lifestyle. Heart disease is the number one cause of death in the United States and is also responsible for tragic disability in millions of Americans. But the vast majority of heart disease is completely avoidable by making some simple lifestyle changes—exercise and upper cervical chiropractic care being the most important.

Everyone knows that exercise is important to a healthy heart and cardiovascular system. But what most people do not realize is how much of an impact the nervous system has on this system as well. The nervous system is responsible for regulating blood flow, heart rate, and blood pressure. Anyone who has experienced a pounding heart during a moment of fright has experienced, first hand, the impact that the nervous system has on the cardiovascular system. In fact, in a recent study published in the *Journal of Human Hypertension*, upper cervical chiropractic adjustments were found to lower the systolic blood pressure by an average of 14 mm Hg in hypertensive patients in comparison to the control group. There was also a decrease in the diastolic blood pressure of an average eight mm Hg as well. The normalizing of blood pressure through upper cervical adjustments has even allowed many people to go off of their blood pressure medication. The authors of this study concluded that the upper cervical adjustments were as effective as the two drug combination therapy.

Immune System

Studying the immune system is like watching a science fiction movie, where amorphous blobs slither around, surrounding and consuming unsuspecting prey. But unlike the science fiction movie where the blobs threaten the existence of human kind, these blobs actually ensure its survival. These blobs are the cells of the immune system. The immune system is a complex army of cells whose sole job is to protect the important cells in the body by eliminating the harmful ones.

Every minute of the day, we are exposed to dangerous bacteria, viruses, fungi, and the development of cancerous cells that, if allowed to grow, would result in illness or death. In fact, the bacteria and viruses in and around our body outnumber the cells that make up our body. Not to mention there is a staggering number or these things in the world around us. They are everywhere. What keeps these invaders in check is the immune system.

When your immune system is compromised due to improper diet, stress, being out of adjustment, or for any other reason, you lose some of your ability to eliminate the harmful cells and invaders in your body, resulting in disease. Just like with your body's other systems, your lifestyle choices have a profound impact on how well your immune system functions.

As with all other systems of the body, the immune system is intimately related to the nervous system. In fact, this relationship is so strong that an entire field of scientific study called psychoneuroimmunology has blossomed to become one of the hottest and most important areas of research. The word, psychoneuroimmunology, refers to the relationship between the mind ("psycho"), the nervous system ("neuro"), and the immune system ("immunology").

Researchers in this field study things like the relationship between emotional stress and cancer and heart disease, how a compromise in the nervous system contributes to immune system abnormalities, and even how infections affect our ability to concentrate. The fundamental property underlying all of this research is the fact that the mind, nervous system, and immune system are like three legs on a stool. If one of them is compromised, the others are affected as well. Therefore, many cases of allergies, autoimmune disorders, and susceptibility to illness are simply the result of a compromised nervous system. Once the nervous system issues are resolved through upper cervical adjustments, the immune system can straighten itself out.

Bones and Joints

The human skeleton is made up of more than 200 bones which are connected by joints. Your bones are responsible for creating your body's general shape, and they serve to protect your internal organs and to manufacture blood cells. Each of your bones is made up of two compounds: a protein meshwork of collagen and a salt of calcium called hydroxyapatite.

The collagen fibers which make up the basic structure of your bones gives them a great deal of resilience and resistance to breaking when twisted, bent, or impacted. It is actually the loss of this collagen meshwork and not just a loss of calcium that is responsible for the bone weakness associated with conditions such as osteoporosis. The other component of bone, hydroxyapatite, is a crystalline calcium salt which is integrated into the collagen meshwork. Hydroxyapatite is responsible for giving the bones rigidity and resistance to crushing under pressure.

Bones can be compared to steel-reinforced concrete, where the collagen meshwork acts much like the steel meshwork in the concrete and the hydroxyapatite acts much like the concrete which surrounds the steel. Together they form a very tough, resilient and rigid framework upon which the rest of the body is supported. But because your bones are rigid and do not bend, you would not be able to move if it were not for your joints.

Joints are much more than simply a place where the ends of two bones meet. They are very complicated systems of ligaments, tendons, membranes, and cartilage that allow the bones to move in a smooth, stable, and controlled way. Joints are designed in a wide variety of ways depending on their function and the particular stresses they have to endure. For example, the joints between your sternum (breastbone) and your ribs are simple joints consisting only of fibrous collagen. They are designed to be simple because the front part of your rib cage does not have to move very much in relation to your sternum. The shoulder joint on the other hand is an extremely complex joint that requires a whole host of muscles, ligaments, and tendons all working in concert with each other in order to move properly. If any one of the muscles or other structures of the shoulder are damaged, pain, instability, or loss of function may result.

Later in this chapter we will discuss a particular set of joints that are especially important; those are the joints of the spine. But first let's take a look at your muscles.

Muscles

There are more than 650 muscles in your body which have only one purpose—to create movement. While your bones are what give your body its framework, it is the muscles that give your body motion. There are more than three times the number of muscles in your body as there are bones, and each one of these muscles fills a particular role in creating movement. Like bones, your muscles also contain a lot of collagen for strength and resilience. But instead of calcium salts, muscles contain a specialized type of cell which has the unique ability to contract when stimulated by the nervous system.

There are actually three types of muscle in the body: smooth muscle, cardiac muscle, and striated muscle (also called skeletal muscle). Smooth muscle is found surrounding the organs of the digestive tract as well as the arteries. In the digestive tract, smooth muscle is responsible for moving the food we eat through our digestive system, while the smooth muscle which surrounds the arteries helps the regulation of blood flow throughout the body. Unlike skeletal muscles, smooth muscles are involuntary muscles, meaning that we do not have conscious control over them.

Cardiac muscle, as its name implies, is found only in the heart. What differentiates cardiac muscle from all other muscle in the body is the fact that it rhythmically contracts on its own, regardless of stimulation by the nervous system. As a matter of fact, if two independent cardiac cells, each rhythmically contracting to their own beat are put in contact with each other, they will begin beating in unison. And it's a good thing, otherwise our heart wouldn't beat very regularly.

The third type of muscle is skeletal muscle. This is the type of muscle that it is responsible for our posture and movement. Every skeletal muscle attaches to at least two different bones and as they contract, they draw the bones together, using the joints as hinges, allowing controlled movement to take place.

Take for example the elbow joint. Compared to some of the other joints in the body, such as the shoulder or hip, the elbow is a relatively simple hinge joint. Yet there are more than a dozen muscles which cross the elbow joint—all of which contribute to the elbow's normal movement. If any of these muscles do not fire in a highly coordinated fashion, or if some of the muscles are tighter than they should be, or if some of the muscles are weaker than they should be, abnormal joint function and pain will likely result. Abnormal posture and joint motion resulting from weak, spasmed, or incoordinated muscles is very common.

Let's continue our discussion of body mechanics by looking at the nervous system.

The Nervous System

The nervous system is made up of trillions of highly-specialized individual nerve cells, each of which communicates with hundreds or thousands of other nerve cells through tiny electrical pulses, and is comprised of two major systems. One is called the central nervous system, which includes your brain and spinal cord, and the other is called the peripheral nervous system, which includes the nerves that run from your spine to all areas of the body. The nervous system is called the master controller as it is responsible for the control of all major body functions including our senses, movement, and balance, as well as the regulations of all body functions.

You experience your life through your nervous system. Everything that you hear, taste, feel, smell, or see filters through your nervous system and is captured and interpreted by your brain. If you see a beautiful sunset and feel good, that is your nervous system. On the other hand, if you see someone crying and feel sad, your nervous system is equally responsible for that experience. Since life as you know it is experienced through your nervous system, it makes sense that you maintain optimal neurological function.

There are four types of nerves that are important to our discussion. These are called pain or sensory nerves, motor nerves, and postural nerves, or more correctly, proprioceptors. The fourth type of nerve is the most important and often the most overlooked and those are the autonomic nerves. The autonomic or "automatic" nerves are vital to the proper function of all of organs and glands.

Pain nerves do just what their name implies—they allow us to feel pain. Whenever something in our body hurts, it is because the pain nerves in the area are being stimulated and sending signals to the brain to create the sensation of pain.

Motor nerves are responsible for controlling our movement by stimulating muscles to contract. The fact that you are able to hold this book in your hands right now is because these motor nerves are contracting the muscles in your hands and arms. If these nerves aren't able to function correctly, it can result in weakness, or even paralysis, in the muscles they control.

The third type of nerve is the proprioceptor, or what we will simply call the postural nerves. These nerves are responsible for sending information to the brain about where your

Your Nervous System

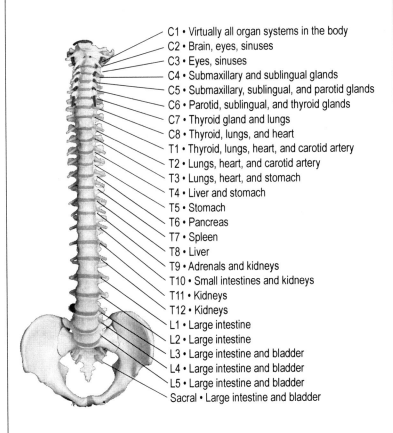

C1 • Virtually all organ systems in the body
C2 • Brain, eyes, sinuses
C3 • Eyes, sinuses
C4 • Submaxillary and sublingual glands
C5 • Submaxillary, sublingual, and parotid glands
C6 • Parotid, sublingual, and thyroid glands
C7 • Thyroid gland and lungs
C8 • Thyroid, lungs, and heart
T1 • Thyroid, lungs, heart, and carotid artery
T2 • Lungs, heart, and carotid artery
T3 • Lungs, heart, and stomach
T4 • Liver and stomach
T5 • Stomach
T6 • Pancreas
T7 • Spleen
T8 • Liver
T9 • Adrenals and kidneys
T10 • Small intestines and kidneys
T11 • Kidneys
T12 • Kidneys
L1 • Large intestine
L2 • Large intestine
L3 • Large intestine and bladder
L4 • Large intestine and bladder
L5 • Large intestine and bladder
Sacral • Large intestine and bladder

All of the functions related to the human body are controlled by the extensive neural network continually sending and receiving electrical impulses to and from the brain. Stress in any part of the nervous system may result in a variety of health problems throughout the body.

body is and what it's doing. For example, if you close your eyes and hold your arm out to your side, you can tell exactly where your arm is even though you can't see it because the postural nerves of the arm and upper back tell the brain where your arm is. Many people have discovered what happens when their postural nerves aren't working correctly after they have had too much to drink. Alcohol partially disrupts your postural nerves, making it difficult to touch your finger to your nose when your eyes are closed, or walk a straight line with your eyes open. When people have interference with the proprioceptor nerves, they often experience a loss of balance or dizziness.

The interesting thing about posture nerves and pain nerves is that they have an opposite relationship. When the posture nerves are working properly we feel less pain. However, if the posture nerves are quiet or interfered with, we experience more pain. An effective way to activate the posture nerves is through movement activities such as exercise. Restoring proper spinal alignment corrects the natural balance between the posture nerves and pain nerves; resulting in decreased pain. Many people in chronic pain have joint misalignment and decreased mobility resulting in chronic pain signals being sent to the brain.

The autonomic nerves "automatically" control the function of the organs and glands. The autonomic nerves are responsible for such things as telling the heart to beat, the stomach to digest, and the immune system to protect. One division of the autonomic nervous system is the sympathetic nervous system, which is responsible for the body's stress response. When the body is under chronic stress as a result of a poor lifestyle, including lack of physical activity, poor diet, and negative thinking, the stress response is initiated.

The stress response is referred to as the "fight or flight" response. The "fight or flight" response has been programmed into our genes since the beginning of time. Its purpose is to protect us from an external threat. Our ancestors, when exposed to a tiger for example, had to either prepare their body for a fight or flee in order to survive. This natural response is intended to be short-lived and results in blood flow to the arms and legs, sugar and cholesterol being delivered to the blood for energy, a narrow state of mental awareness, and a decrease in immune function. Nowadays, we are not threatened by tigers but instead mortgages, relationships, bosses, environmental chemicals, and sedentary lifestyles. Instead of the stress response being short-lived, it is often turned on for days, weeks, months, or years resulting in disease. In fact, the result of chronic stress stimulation is high sugar, high cholesterol, high blood pressure, immune suppression, fat deposits, muscle spasm, and fatigue. Most of today's chronic illnesses can be attributed to the chronic stress response which is all part of the autonomic nervous system.

The other half of the autonomic nervous system is called the parasympathetic nervous system, which has the opposite effect of the sympathetic nervous system; it creates the "feed or breed" response. This is the part of the nervous system that is responsible for the relaxed feeling that you feel after a good meal or when you sit around with a loved one. The body should naturally be operating in this state. This is when the body is able to heal, grow, and repair itself. There are effective wellness tools and methods to help turn off the "fight or flight" response and turn on the healthy "feed or breed" response. These include gentle chiropractic care, meditation, yoga, Pilates, prayer, massage, taking a bubble bath, or even doing something you enjoy such as golf, a hobby, or dinner with your loved one.

The chiropractic adjustment has the ability to balance the nervous system and is one of the most effective, least expensive, and healthiest ways to activate the parasympathetic nervous system. Our ability to be healthy and well will directly depend upon us adopting healthier lifestyle habits. Better health through better chemistry has failed, better health through better lifestyle is the answer.

The Three Pillars of Body Mechanics

As we have discussed in the previous sections of this chapter, the human body is an amazingly complex system of bones, joints, muscles, and nerves, designed to work together to accomplish one thing: movement. Movement is one of the defining characteristics that separates us from plants, bacteria, and fungus. Everything about the human body is designed with movement in mind—nerve fibers stimulate the muscles to contract, muscles contract to move the bones, bones move around joints, and the nervous system controls it all.

Movement or exercise is not a therapy to fix something or an optional activity; it is the most essential nutrient for the brain. As a matter of fact, research has shown that movement is so critical to our body's health that a lack of movement has a detrimental affect on everything from digestion, to our emotional state, immune function, our ability to concentrate, how well we sleep, and even to how long we live. The bottom line is that if your lifestyle does not include enough movement, your body cannot function efficiently. Consequently, three things will happen: first, you will not be as physically healthy and will suffer from a wide variety of physical ailments, ranging from headaches to high blood pressure. Second, you will not be as productive in your life because of reduced energy levels and the ability to mentally focus. Third, because you have less energy, your activity level will tend to drop off even further over time, creating a downward spiral of reduced energy and less activity until you get to a point where even the demands of a sedentary job leave you physically exhausted by the end of the day.

Pillar One: Posture

The ancient Japanese art form of growing Bonsai trees is fascinating. They are essentially normal shrubs that have been consistently stressed in a particular way for a long time to create a posture which would never be found in nature. Depending on how the tree is stressed while it grows, it may end up looking like a miniature version of a full-sized tree, or it may end up looking like a wild tangle of branches with twists and loops. Every day in my practice, I see the human equivalent of Bonsai trees walk through my door—people with an unnatural posture due to the continual daily stresses on their body.

The most immediate problem with poor posture is that it creates a lot of chronic muscle tension as the weight of the head and upper body is having to be supported by the muscles instead of the bones. This effect becomes more pronounced the further your posture deviates from your Structural Center (See illustration).

To illustrate this idea further, think about carrying a briefcase. If you had to carry your briefcase with your arms outstretched in front of you, it would not take long before the muscles of your shoulders would be completely exhausted. This is because carrying the briefcase far away from your Structural Center places an undue stress on your shoulder muscles. If you held the same briefcase down at your side, your muscles would not fatigue as quickly because the briefcase is closer to your Structural Center and the weight is, therefore, supported by the bones of the skeleton, rather than the muscles.

In some parts of the world, women can carry big pots full of water from distant water sources back to their homes. They are able to carry these heavy pots a long distance without significant effort because they balance them on the top of their heads, thereby carrying them at their Structural Center and allowing the strength of their skeleton to bear the weight, rather than their muscles.

Correcting poor posture and the physical problems that result are accomplished by doing two things. The first is to eliminate as much 'bad' stress from your body as possible. Bad stress includes all the factors, habits or stressors that cause your body to deviate from your Structural Center.

The second is to apply 'good' stress on the body in an effort to move your posture back toward your Structural Center. Getting your body back to its Structural Center by improving your posture is critically important to improving how you feel.

Your Structural Center

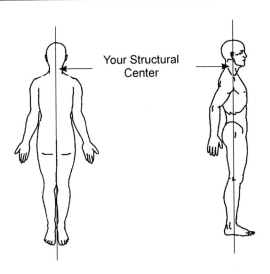

Your Structural Center

Your Structural Center is the imaginary line that runs through your body where all of the forces are perfectly balanced and supported by your skeleton, rather than your muscles.

Pillar Two: Mobility

Imagine waking up one morning with a frozen shoulder where you couldn't move your upper arm more than a few inches in any direction. How much would that impact your ability to do your job? How much would that affect your ability to drive your car or even to dress yourself? How much would that affect your ability to concentrate on anything other than your shoulder? Obviously, if your shoulder did not move correctly, it would have a dramatic impact on your life. Well, the same is true with mobility in every part of your body. If things aren't moving the way they are supposed to move, it will have a negative impact on your ability to function at work, take care of the demands of everyday life and even your ability to concentrate.

Over the years, I have had a number of patients come into my office with severe low back pain who stated that their pain came on suddenly when they did something as simple as bend down to pet their cat, put on their socks, or pick up the newspaper. Just about everyone would agree that a person's body should be able to handle something as simple as bending over to pick up a newspaper or putting on their socks, right? So what happened?

In every one of these cases, we found that many of the joints in their body were barely moving at all; they were 'all locked up.' When the joints in one area of the body do not move the way they should, other areas of the body are forced to move more than they were designed to in an effort to compensate for the area that is not moving. This creates a significant stress on the areas that are having to pick up the slack of the joints that aren't moving so well. This soon leads to pain and inflammation. At the same time, the areas that don't have normal movement will slowly worsen as the muscles continue to tighten, the joints stick together and the ligaments and tendons shorten. This lack of mobility and improper alignment leads to progressive wear and tear and the degenerative or arthritic process begins.

Just as the teeth can decay without proper dental hygiene, the spine will decay as a result of improper spinal hygiene. Spinal hygiene consists of daily spinal movement, proper ergonomics, and proper alignment and spinal function. Spinal decay is irreversible so the early adoption of a spinal hygiene routine is essential to proper prevention of future spinal problems. Spinal decay leaves the body in a very unstable condition and if left unchecked, this process will continue until the body can hardly move at all and the person suffers flare-ups of pain at the slightest provocation.

Most of us have seen people who have lost most of their normal mobility; they look like their whole body has been starched stiff whenever they try to move around. This is especially prevalent among the elderly. Contrary to popular belief, this is not the inevitable effect of aging, rather it is the inevitable effect of not maintaining the body's mobility and alignment through exercise, stretching, and upper cervical chiropractic care. There are a lot of people in their 60s, 70s, and beyond, who are stronger and more flexible than the average person in their 30s simply because they keep themselves exercising. Maintaining mobility and alignment is critical in order to live free from pain and disability. Maintaining good mobility is not difficult, but it does not happen on its own.

Just as in developing a good posture, it is necessary that you exercise and stretch to keep your muscles, ligaments, and tendons flexible and healthy. In addition, it is necessary that all of the joints in your body are kept moving correctly as well through proper alignment. Flexibility is a sign of health. The healthiest populations in our society are the most flexible; the newborn and the elite athlete have the most mobility in their joints. Most people find upper cervical chiropractic care to be a safe, gentle, and effective way to improve their posture and flexibility.

Pillar Three: Strength

Strong muscles keep your body upright and allow you to move. Good muscle strength and balance are critical for proper posture and to minimize muscle tension. Your muscles function much like the wires that hold up a tall radio or television antenna. If the wires are equally strong on all sides, the antenna will stand up straight. If one of the wires becomes weak or breaks, the antenna will either lean to the side or collapse. The same is true with your body. If the muscles on all sides of your spine are balanced and strong, your body will stand up straight and strong. Unfortunately, most people don't have balanced and strong muscles. The reason for this gets back to exercise and alignment.

Muscles are very efficient at getting stronger or weaker in response to the demands placed on them. Since most of us sit at a desk, drive a car, and sit on the sofa at home, many of our muscles are not challenged. Consequently, they become weak. At the same time, the muscles that are constantly used throughout the day become strong. This imbalance of muscle strength contributes to poor posture and chronic muscle tension. Left unchecked, muscle imbalances tend to get worse, not better, because of a phenomenon called *reciprocal inhibition.*

Reciprocal inhibition literally means "shutting down the opposite." Simply put, for all of the muscles that move your body in one direction, there are opposing muscles that move the body in the opposite direction. In order to keep these muscles from working against each other, when the body contracts one muscle group, it forces the opposing group to relax—it shuts down the opposite muscles.

Restoring alignment will correct the neurological distur-bances that are responsible for imbalanced and weakend muscles.

The Mechanics of Your Spine

Now that you are an expert on all of the major aspects of body mechanics and you understand why it is so important that the skeletal system, muscular system, and nervous system work together in a tightly coordinated way, let's take a look at the single-most complex and important system of bones, muscles and nerves in your body—your spine.

Your spine is one of the most complex systems in the body, consisting of nearly a hundred intricate joints and trillions of nerve pathways connected together by a complicated meshwork of ligaments, tendons, cartilage, and muscles. The spine is designed to do three things simultaneously: 1) protect the spinal cord that serves as the primary communication conduit between your brain and the rest of your body; 2) serve as a structural support upon which all of your organs and upper body rests; and 3) provide an incredible amount of mobility and flexibility, allowing you to bend forward to touch your toes, swim, throw a baseball, and turn your head. Unfortunately, with this degree of mobility and flexibility comes instability—the susceptibility to misalignment and injury.

In order to function correctly, all of the bones, joints, muscles, and nerves have to work in perfect coordination in order to maintain your proper posture, strength, and movement. A disruption in the position or movement in any one of the bones of the spine or a loss of muscle balance or coordination will impose a significant stress on the spine.

Fortunately, most of us don't experience a severe problem with our spine or spinal cord, but small problems occur all the time. These happen when we slip and fall, are in a car accident, sleep in a strange bed, sit with poor posture, "throw our back out" from shoveling snow from the driveway, or lift something incorrectly. It's typically not just injury to the bones and joints themselves that causes problems in the spine. Damage to the muscles and connective tissue are just as important, for these are the structures that are responsible for supporting the bones and joints. Once these tissues are damaged, the vertebrae can lose their correct alignment or movement. When this happens, it not only can cause pain and loss of function in the back, but also can affect the other areas of the body.

Let's review the basic construction of the spine. The spine is made up of a stacked set of bones called the vertebrae. These are like the bricks upon which our entire structure is built. Each vertebra consists of a vertebral body, that is a large oval-shaped solid block of bone, and a vertebral arch, which is located on the back of the vertebral body and creates the space through which the spinal cord runs.

Each vertebra is attached to two adjacent spinal vertebrae, with a disc between them. These discs, technically called inter-vertebral discs, are thick pads of fibrocartilage that act as shock absorbers and give the spine its ability to flex and twist. The disc itself is kind of like jelly-filled Danish. It has an outer fibrous portion called the annulus, and a soft jelly-like center called the nucleus pulposus.

A disc herniation occurs when the fibers in one portion of the annulus are torn allowing the nucleus pulposus to partially push through the annulus, creating a bulge in the outer disc; much like a tire develops a bulge when there is a break in one of the underlying supporting fibers. Disc bulges do not always lead to pain, but quite often they do. The pain may come from the irritation of the nerves within the disc itself, or it may be caused by the disc bulge impinging upon a nerve that runs through the area. As we age, our discs tend to dehydrate and break down. This process is accelerated by smoking and not keeping yourself fully hydrated, as well as by a sedentary lifestyle, including poor posture, and lack of joint alignment and mobility.

Between each pair of vertebrae and behind the disc, there is a small space where the nerves exit from the spinal cord and run to all of the areas of the body. This space is called the vertebral foramen. Foramen is an impressive medical term that simply means "hole." Vertebral foramina (holes) can become compressed when a disc bulge presses into the area, if inflammation causes the tissues in the area to swell, or if the intervertebral disc becomes dehydrated. When this happens, excruciating pain can result which radiates to other areas of the body.

Ligaments bind the vertebra together and tendons attach numerous muscles to each segment. These ligaments and tendons help to absorb shock and to restrict how much movement there is between each set of spinal vertebrae. Unfortunately, these ligaments and tendons can be damaged whenever spinal vertebrae are forcefully moved beyond their normal limits— such as in a whiplash or sports injury. An injury to a ligament is called a sprain. If the injury is to the tendon or muscle, it is referred to as a strain.

Muscles attach to the bony extensions of the vertebra and provide movement in the spine by contracting in a highly coordinated way. Like ligaments, muscles are important for absorbing shock and releasing it in a controlled way. For example, when your heel strikes the ground as you walk it is your muscles that abate the shock before it reaches your head so that your teeth don't clatter together each time you take a step.

As a whole, the spine forms the protective housing for the spinal cord, which begins at the brain stem (back of the skull) and extends like a wire down the length of the spine. Ultimately, the spinal cord sends out nerve branches that send and receive signals from every cell in the body. The close relationship between the spine and the spinal cord means that damage to any of the discs or vertebrae can also affect the spine or the spinal nerves associated with it, causing pain or abnormal function of the structures innervated by the affected area.

The spine is divided into four different regions. The upper seven vertebrae in the neck are collectively called the "cervical spine," with the skull sitting directly upon the first cervical vertebra. The most vital area of the spine is located at the top of the neck. The top vertebrae in the neck is also known as the Atlas or C1. It is called the Atlas because it holds up the skull, just as the Greek god, Atlas held up the world. The majority of our neck's motion occurs between the Atlas and the Axis vertebrae. The Axis, or C2, is the second vertebrae in the neck. It is called the Axis because the Atlas, a donut shaped bone, rotates around it. These bones protect the top of spinal cord which sits below the brainstem, the area where the brain meets the spinal cord. Most vital functions of the body are controlled at the level of the brainstem including cardiac, respiratory, vascular, immune, and postural functions. As a direct result of the degree of mobility of these two vertebrae, they are also the most unstable and consequently, are the most likely to become misaligned. The upper cervical misalignment or subluxation can affect the entire nervous system, and therefore can affect all of the systems of the body.

The middle twelve vertebrae are called the "thoracic vertebrae." All of the thoracic vertebrae have a pair of ribs attached to them. The twelve pair of ribs are important for protecting several of your internal organs and are critical for breathing. The lower five vertebrae are referred to as the "lumbar vertebrae" and because of the fact that they bear the full weight of your upper body, are the most frequently injured. The lowest region of the spine is called the sacrum. During childhood the sacrum is made up of five vertebrae, just like the lumbar spine. During later childhood, these five vertebrae fuse together to make one solid bone called the sacrum. Technically speaking, kids have six more bones in their spine than adults do.

When viewed from the front or back, the spine should appear perfectly straight and symmetrical, reflecting the fact that your body is also symmetrical when viewed from the front or back. When viewed from the side, however, four major curves should be seen—one in each of the cervical, thoracic, lumbar and sacral regions. In both the cervical and lumbar regions of the spine, the curves bend backward. These are called "lordotic" curves. The curves in the thoracic and sacral regions bend forward. These are called "kyphotic" curves. As strange as it may seem, these curves actually add a considerable amount of strength and resiliency to the spine. Think about the curves as being like a spring, allowing the spine to flex and absorb shock much better than if it were straight. In fact, when a region of the spine loses its normal curve, as often happens in the neck following a whiplash injury or consistent and persistent microtrauma, the discs that separate the vertebrae begin to degenerate.

Because of the complexity and instability of the spine and its potential for affecting so many systems in the body, this is the structure that chiropractors end up working on more than anything else. Chiropractors are more than back doctors; they are also nerve doctors. The chiropractor only uses the spine to access and influence the central nervous system which as you now know is located and protected by the spine.

Problems in the spine can come from a variety of sources:

- *Discs can become herniated and compress nerves that go to the legs or arms.*
- *The joints between the vertebrae may become stuck.*
- *The bones, ligaments, or joints themselves may be injured.*
- *The disc space itself can be a source of pain.*
- *The muscles surrounding the spine may become injured.*
- *Muscle spasms may develop due to overuse or injury.*
- *Inflammation from overuse, injury, or disease may irritate the spine.*

Quick Review

We covered a whole lot of stuff in this chapter. Let's review quickly before moving on. We discussed the four components

The Regions of Your Spine

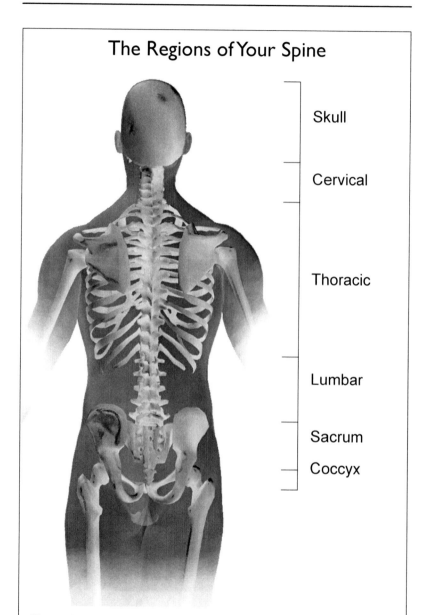

Skull

Cervical

Thoracic

Lumbar

Sacrum

Coccyx

Your spine is comprised of five regions. These are the cervical (neck region), the thoracic (mid back region), the lumbar (low back region), the sacrum and the coccyx (tailbone).

of the neuromusculoskeletal system; the bones and joints which serve as the framework for the body, the muscles which are responsible for movement and the nervous system which is responsible for controlling it all. We discussed the Three Pillars of Body Mechanics—posture, mobility, and strength—and why each of these are important.

You learned that when your posture deviates from your Structural Center, your muscles tighten up, resulting in nerve pressure, pain, and decreased mobility. You learned that once you begin to lose mobility and alignment, it usually continues to worsen unless you restore your spinal alignment and re-establish normal motion. You learned about the central role that the nervous system plays in the stress response and organ system function. You learned that muscles will either become stronger or weaker depending on how much they get used, and that muscular imbalances will often lead to chronic muscle spasms and pain. Finally, you learned that your spine is an incredibly complex and important structure for your overall health due to its close relationship to the spinal cord. If any of the structures of the spine are injured or are not functioning correctly, pain or disability is the result. More importantly as the structures of the spine become misaligned they will have a devastating effect on the central nervous system which will always result in decreased health and dis-ease.

It is important to remember that you live your life through your nervous system; it is therefore important to keep it as healthy as possible.

3

An Introduction to Chiropractic

The word "chiropractic" comes from the Greek words *cheir* (hand) and *praxis* (action) and literally means "done by hand." Instead of prescribing drugs or performing surgeries, chiropractors choose to use manual corrections of the spine and joints, and lifestyle coaching to stimulate and entice the body's natural (innate) state of health to fully express itself.

Similar to conventional medicine, chiropractic is based upon scientific principles of (1) assessment through testing and empirical observation and (2) intervention and care based upon the practitioner's rigorous training and clinical experience. But unlike conventional medicine, that tends to focus on treating disease symptoms once they occur, chiropractic focuses on improving the health of the individual in an effort to avoid illness in the first place. Most people would rather be healthy and avoid illness, if they could. This is one of the main reasons for the big surge in the popularity of chiropractic. People are recognizing the benefit of seeking an alternative to traditional medicine; one that will help them achieve optimal health and create wellness in their lives.

So, what is health? Most people have adopted the belief that they are healthy when they feel good, but this is only part of the story. According to the Dorland's Medical Dicitionary, health is a complete state of mental, physical, and social wellbeing and not merely the absence of disease or infirmity. This definition does not mention that "feeling good" is a requirement for health.

The reality is that symptoms have very little to do with health. Just consider some of the major diseases like heart disease, cancer, stroke, diabetes, hypertension, AIDS, and osteoporosis. These are some of the worst conditions that the body can suffer, yet most people who have these conditions never have an inkling that they are sick until the diseases are in their advanced stages. In fact, the first symptom of advanced heart disease is sometimes a life-threating heart attack!

Many people are walking around with these states of ill health right now and they don't know it because they are under the misperception that since they are not suffering any pain, they are healthy. On the other hand, how much does the excruciating pain of a stubbed toe tell us about our overall health? Not much.

"If I am not 'sick' then I am healthy" is another false belief. Think about this for a moment: there is a big difference between "not poor" and "rich," or "not dumb" and "smart." There is an equally big difference between "not sick" and "healthy." Not feeling sick does not equal health, yet so many people are settling for it and believing that they are healthy. I contest that there is a is a large difference between "not sick" and "healthy." The belief that "symptoms equals a health problem," and the belief that by using medication to alleviate symptoms you are healthy is perpetuated by our culture, which relies heavily on a medical, media, and pharmaceutical machine that makes money when people take pills.

Too often, the medicine is only successful at simply masking the symptom, not correcting the disease process itself. The person taking the medication is left with the false impression that they have taken the appropriate action, when in fact, their body has been left in its unhealthy state and simply continues on the same course of ill health.

Are all symptoms bad? Not at all. Symptoms, such as pain, serve as a way for the body to communicate to us that we are not living right. Consider the scenario of a person who makes some poor lifestyle choices in the form of poor diet, lack of exercise, and poor stress management. As a result of this unhealthy lifestyle, they live in a constant state of stress and deficiency in the essential nutritional components that the body requires and their immune system suffers because of it. This reduced resistance from a compromised immune system then allows bacteria, which are always present in our bodies, to grow unchecked and illness results. Even more dangerous is the fact that when the immune system is compromised, it no longer is as effective at fighting off cancer and other more dangerous conditions.

In our practice, we define health as the state when 100 percent of the body parts are functioning at 100 percent, 100 percent of the time. This means that: first, we must have 100 percent of our body parts. If in the unfortunate circumstance that we lost one of our parts or had one removed there is very little we can do about that now. Since nature does not endow us with spare parts, the loss of any part of our body will, by definition, have some negative impact on our overall functioning—at least to some degree.

Second, our goal is to be functioning at 100 percent in the present time. While we cannot do anything about the time that has passed, we can do a lot to make sure that we have optimal health today. The only time that we can impact is right here in the present, and this will, in turn, directly shape our health in the future. In fact, it is the health choices earlier in life that have led people to their current state of health. Likewise, it will be the choices that are made from this point on that will determine one's health destiny.

The last component of this definition is function. Function is the key to health. When our body is functioning at its peak capacity we are truly healthy.

What system of the body controls the function of the

body? The answer is the nervous system. As we dicussed in the previous chapter, the brain and the spinal cord make up the central nervous system which is responsible for the control and coordination of every cell, organ, and tissue of the body. If the nervous system is responsible for our function, healing, growth, and repair then it is imperative that people should be aware of the health status of their nervous system. It also make sense that people should make sure that their nervous system is functioning at its peak capacity.

This is where chiropractors fit into the wellness lifestyle. Chiropractors are spine and nervous system experts. We understand that one of the main causes of pain and dis-ease is the misalignment and abnormal motion of the vertebrae in the spinal column. Misalignment of the spine negatively impacts an individual's healing and repair because it interferes with the central nervous system. If there was something interfering with your nervous system, would you be healthier or sicker? Sicker of course. Chiropractors remove nervous system interference by adjusting the spine, thereby relieving pressure and irritation on the nerves, restoring joint mobility, and returning the body back to a state of normal function.

Numerous studies have demonstrated that chiropractic care is one of the most effective approaches for people who suffer with back pain, neck pain, headaches, whiplash, fatigue, sports injuries, and many other types of neuromusculoskeletal problems. Chiropractic does not cure these diseases but instead enables people with these symptoms to recover their health naturally by removing interference with the nervous system and the body's natural healing response. Many people are unaware that chiropractic has been effective for people with high blood pressure, fibromyalgia, multiple sclerosis and children with ear infections (otitis media), asthma and neurodevelopmental/ behavioral disorders.

Health care can be divided into two approaches: *mechanistic* and *vitalistic*. The *mechanistic* approach is very reductionistic. Mechanism attempts to understand how each part of the body works, down to its smallest unit, the cell. Then, the mechanistic logic attempts to intervene with the part of the body that seems to not be working in an attempt to make that part work again. This is usually undertaken with medication. If the medication is not effective in making the part work again, then the part may be removed by surgery.

The limitation of this health care model is that it does not recognize the interrelatedness of the body parts. A doctor cannot intervene with one part of the body with out affecting all of the other parts of the body. The interconnectedness of the body is the reason why there are so many side effects when one takes a medication to treat one part of the body.

Chiropractic health care is *vitalistic*, meaning that it addresses your overall health. What is the difference between a living human being and a dead body? All the parts are the same. I am confident that most people would recognize that there is something animating the living body but not the dead body. Some people may call it energy, chi, spirit, nature, god, or the more scientific explanation would be electrical current. In chiropractic, this life energy and animation is referred to as *innate intelligence.*

The vitalistic approach toward health care recognizes that the body has an inborn wisdom or innate intelligence that runs the body and promotes healing. Think about it—you do not have to tell your lungs to breathe, your stomach to digest, or your heart to beat. Instead, these processes of self-regulation are controlled by your nervous system. Likewise, the body has an inborn potential to heal itself. When you cut your finger or break a bone, what makes new skin or new bone? This is accomplished by the body's wisdom, not the Band-Aid or the cast.

Our potential to regain and improve our health will directly depend on our ability to invoke and inspire our innate intelligence. The good news is health is the natural state of the body. Being sick and ill is not natural. Through scientific chiropractic care and proper lifestyle choices the body's inborn wisdom can be stoked, fueled, and turned on to promote healing and the recovery of your natural state: health.

I recognize that many lifestyle factors such as exercise, diet, rest, and your environment impact your health. For this reason, I always recommend changes in lifestyle—eating, exercise, thinking well, and improved sleeping habits—in addition to chiropractic care.

The History of Chiropractic

Manual manipulation of the spine and other joints in the body have been around for a long time. Ancient writings from China and Greece dating between 2700 BC and 1500 BC mention spinal manipulation and the maneuvering of the lower extremities to ease low back pain. In fact, Hippocrates, the famous Greek physician who lived from 460 to 357 BC, published a text detailing the importance of manual manipulation. In one of his writings he declares, "Get knowledge of the spine, for this is the requisite for many diseases." Evidence of manual manipulation of the body has been found among the ancient civilizations of Egypt, Babylon, Syria, Japan, the Incas, Mayans, and Native Americans.

The official beginning of the chiropractic profession dates back to 1895 when Daniel David Palmer restored the hearing of Harvey Lillard by manually adjusting his neck, and something told him that he was into something good. Two years later, in 1897, Dr. Palmer went on to begin the Palmer School of Chiropractic in Davenport, Iowa, which continues to train doctors of chiropractic to this day.

Throughout the twentieth century, the profession of chiropractic has gained considerable recognition and scientific support. Research studies that have clearly demonstrated the value of chiropractic care in reducing health care costs, improving recovery rates and increasing patient satisfaction. In fact, one very large study conducted in Canada, the 1993 Manga Study, concluded that chiropractic care would save hundreds of millions of dollars annually in work disability payments and direct health care costs. Several major studies conducted by the U.S. Government, the Rand Corporation, and others, have all demonstrated the incredible value of chiropractic care. Unfortunately, there are still many people who have never been to a chiropractor and don't understand what we do. My hope is that this book will help educate more people about this wonderful field of health care.

The Vertebral Subluxation Complex

What truly differentiates doctors of chiropractic from any other health care professionals is the fact that chiropractors are the only professionals who are trained to detect and correct what are called spinal *subluxations.* The word "subluxation" comes from the Latin words meaning "to dislocate" (luxare) and "somewhat or slightly" (sub). So the term "vertebral subluxation" literally means a slight dislocation (misalignment) of the bones in the spine.

Although this term was adequate in the 1800s when much was still misunderstood about the human body, today the word "subluxation" has changed in meaning to capture the complex of neurological, structural, and functional changes that occur when a bone is "out of place." For this reason chiropractors usually refer to subluxations of the spine as the "vertebral subluxation complex," or "VSC" for short. There are actually five components that contribute to the vertebral subluxation complex (VSC). They are:

1) The bone component, where the vertebrae are either out of position, not moving properly, or are undergoing degeneration.

This frequently leads to a narrowing of the spaces between the bones through which the nerves pass; often resulting in irritation or impingement of the nerve itself.

2) The nervous component. This includes the disruption of the normal flow of energy along the nerve fibers, causing the messages traveling along the nerves to become distorted. The result is that all of the tissues that are fed by those nerves receive distorted signals from the brain and, consequently, are not able to function normally. Over time, this can lead to a whole host of conditions, such as peptic ulcers, constipation, and other organ system dysfunction. When nerve energy is disrupted as it flows from the body up to the brain, it results in a loss of balance, uncoordination of movement, cognitive changes, emotional changes, poor posture, and a suppressed immune system.

3) The muscular component. Since nerves control the muscles that help hold the vertebrae in place, muscles have to be considered to be an integral part of the vertebral subluxation complex. In fact, muscles both affect, and are affected by the VSC. A subluxation can irritate a nerve, the irritated nerve can cause a muscle to spasm, the spasmed muscle pulls the attached vertebrae further out of place, which then further irritates the nerve, and you have a vicious cycle. It is no wonder that very few subluxations just go away by themselves.

4) The soft tissue component. The VSC will also affect the surrounding tendons, ligaments, blood supply, and other tissues as the misaligned vertebrae tug and squeeze the connective tissue with tremendous force. Over time, the soft tissues can become stretched out or scarred, leaving the spine with either a permanent instability or restriction.

5) The chemical component is the change in the chemistry of the body due to the VSC. Most often, the chemical changes, such as the release of a class of chemicals called "kinins," are pro-inflammatory; meaning that they increase inflammation in the affected area.

These changes get progressively worse over time if they are not treated correctly, leading to chronic pain, inflammation, arthritis, muscle trigger points, the formation of bone spurs, loss of movement, as well as muscle weakness and spasm. Chiropractors have known the dangers of the vertebral subluxation complex ever since the birth of the profession. More and more scientific research is demonstrating the tremendous detrimental impact that subluxations have on the tissue of the body. In order to be truly healthy, it is vital that your nervous system be functioning free of interference from subluxations. Chiropractors are the only health professionals trained in the detection, location, and correction of the vertebral subluxation complex through chiropractic care.

Chiropractic Care

Spinal adjustments to correct subluxations are what makes doctors of chiropractic unique in comparison with any other type of health care professional. The term "adjustment" refers to the specific manipulation chiropractors apply to vertebrae that have abnormal movement patterns or fail to function normally. The objective of the chiropractic care is to reduce the subluxation, which results in an increased range of motion, reduced nerve irritability, and improved function.

Not all chiropractors and chiropractic techniques are the same. Some chiropractic techniques rely on quick thrusts applied to a vertebra for the purpose of correcting its position, movement or both. These adjustments are the type that most people associate with chiropractic care. However, there are many chiropractic techniques that do not rely on twisting and turning the body, and forceful adjustments. These techniques are referred to as low-force chiropractic techniques.

Low-force techniques enable the chiropractor to apply a gentle yet specific input into the spine that is usually very comfortable for the patient. These techniques although very subtle, are very powerful. They directly influence the body's highest control centers, the brain and spinal cord.

Chiropractic is so much more than simply a means of relieving pain. Ultimately, the goal of the chiropractic care is to restore the body to its natural state of optimal health. Since the body has a remarkable ability to heal itself and to maintain its own health, my primary focus is simply to remove those things which interfere with the body's normal healing ability.

As mentioned, chiropractors understand that within each of us is an innate wisdom, a health energy, that will express itself as perfect health and well-being if we simply allow it to. Therefore, the focus of chiropractic care is simply to remove any physiological blocks to the proper expression of the body's innate wisdom. Once these subluxations are removed, health is the natural consequence.

The Three Phases of Chiropractic Care

Chiropractic care following an injury is like building a house—certain things have to happen in a particular order in order for everything to stand strong and work the way it is supposed to. If you tried to put up your walls before you had a solid foundation, your walls would be weak and eventually collapse. If you tried to put on your roof before the walls were ready, you would run into the same problem. The same is true for your body. Your body has to go through a particular plan of care in order to repair itself correctly and fully. There are three general phases of chiropractic care; 1) relief care, 2) corrective care, and, 3) wellness care.

Phase One—Relief Care

Many people go to a chiropractor because they are in pain. In this first phase of care, the main goal is to relieve your symptoms and to begin making the desired changes to the spine and nervous system. Sometimes this will require frequent visits.

Most people are under the assumption that if they don't feel any pain that there is nothing wrong with them – that they are healthy. Unfortunately, pain is a very poor indicator of health. In fact, pain and other symptoms frequently only appear after a disease or other condition has become advanced. For example, consider a cavity in your tooth. Does it hurt when it first develops or after it has become serious? Regardless of whether you are talking about cancer, heart disease, diabetes, stress or problems with the spine, pain is usually the last thing to appear. When you begin chiropractic care, pain is also the first symptom to disappear, even though much of the underlying condition remains.

The Three Phases of Chiropractic Care

Phase 1	Phase 2	Phase 3
Relief Care	**Corrective Care**	**Wellness Care**
The first objective is to relieve pain and begin to make changes to your spine and nervous system.	During the corrective care phase, muscles, nerves, and other tissues are allowed to heal more completely, thereby helping to prevent re-injury.	Once your body has fully healed, it is important to come in for periodic adjustments to improve your well-being as an integral part of a healthy lifestyle.

Phase Two—Corrective Care

Most chiropractors regard the elimination of symptoms as the easiest part of a course of care. If all that the chiropractor does is to remove the pain and stop there, the chances of the condition recurring are much greater. In order to avoid a rapid recurrence of symptoms, it is necessary to continue care even though your symptoms are gone. Often, the symptoms will disappear long before the problem (subluxation) is corrected.

During the correction phase of your care, you will not have to be adjusted as often as you were during the first phase of care and, depending on your particular circumstances, you may begin doing exercises and stretches at home to help accelerate your healing. It is during this crucial phase of care that your spine will be strengthened and surrounding tissues will begin to stabilize and heal. Correcting the surrounding soft tissues is essential to achieve a recovery.

Treatment during the corrective phase helps to minimize the likelihood of your symptoms returning. Do not be discouraged if you have mild flare-ups in your symptoms on occasion. This is normal. Flare-ups are bound to occur during the corrective phase because your body has not fully recovered. Depending on the severity of your injury or condition and how long you have been suffering from it, this phase of your care may last anywhere from a few months to a couple of years.

Phase Three—Wellness Care

Many chiropractic patients, once they see the impact that the care has had on their activities of daily living, come to the conclusion that chiropractic care is a beneficial aspect of an active healthy lifestyle. Much like people choose to exercise and eat right for life, many people choose to incorporate regular chiropractic care into their wellness regimen. Once your body has fully healed, routine wellness chiropractic care can help to ensure that your physical problems do not return and helps keep your body in optimal condition. Just like continuing an exercise program and eating well in order to sustain the benefits of exercise and proper diet, it is necessary to continue chiropractic care to ensure the health of your nervous system and, in turn, your entire body. When you make routine chiropractic care a part of your lifestyle, you avoid many of the aches and pains that so many people suffer though, your joints will last longer and you will be able to engage in more of the activities you love.

The Myths and Facts about Chiropractic

As successful as chiropractic has become, there are a lot of myths about chiropractic floating around in the general public. Times have definitely changed for the better, but the fact is that many people still do not understand what chiropractors do. Let's talk about a few of the more common myths about chiropractic.

Myth: Chiropractors are not real doctors.

Chiropractors are licensed as primary health care providers in every U.S. state and dozens of countries around the world. The chiropractic and medical school curricula are virtually identical. In fact, chiropractors have more hours of education than their medical counterparts. As part of their education, chiropractic students also complete approximately nine hundred hours of work in a clinical setting, assisting licensed chiropractors. Once chiropractic students graduate, they have to pass four sets of national board exams as well as state board exams in the states they want to practice.

Chiropractors receive extensive training, combined with many hours of practical work. Just like conventional medical doctors, chiropractors are primary care professionals that are subject to the same testing, licensing and monitoring by state and national peer-reviewed boards. Federal and state programs, such as Medicare, Medicaid, and Workers' Compensations programs cover chiropractic, and all federal agencies accept sick-leave certificates signed by doctors of chiropractic.

The biggest difference between chiropractors and medical doctors lies not in their education or diagnostic ability, but in their preferred method of care. Medical doctors are trained in the use of medicines (chemicals that affect your internal biochemistry) and surgery. Chiropractors are trained in adjusting, nutrition, exercise and wellness care—the core essentials for an active healthy life.

Myth: Medical doctors don't like chiropractors.

The American Medical Association's opposition to chiropractic was at its strongest in the 1940s under the leadership of Morris Fishbein. Fishbein called chiropractors "rabid dogs" and referred to them as "playful and cute, but killers." He tried to portray chiropractors as members of an unscientific cult, caring about nothing but taking their patients' money. Up until the late 1970s and early 1980s, the medical establishment purposely conspired to try to destroy the profession of chiropractic. In fact, a landmark lawsuit in the 1980s found that the American Medical Association was guilty of conspiracy, and the Association was ordered to pay restitution.

In the twenty years since then, the position of most medical doctors has changed; mostly because of several major studies that showed the superiority of chiropractic in treating a host of conditions, coupled with a better understanding among medical doctors about what chiropractors actually do. Many hospitals across the country now have chiropractors on staff and many chiropractic offices have medical doctors on staff. Chiropractors and medical doctors are now much more comfortable working together in cases where medical care is necessary as an adjunct to chiropractic care.

*Myth: Once you start going to a chiropractor,
you have to keep going the rest of your life.*

This is a statement that I frequently hear when the topic of chiropractic care comes up in conversation. This statement is only partly true. You only have to continue going to the chiropractor as long as you wish to maintain the health of your neuro-musculoskeletal system. Going to a chiropractor is much like going to the dentist, exercising at a gym or eating a healthier diet, as long as you keep it up, you continue to enjoy the benefits. People who choose to use chiropractic care on an ongoing basis are not doing so because they have to. Instead, they have seen the impact and the benefits that chiropractic care has had on their life and they choose to utilize chiropractic services as part of a healthy lifestyle.

Many years ago, dentists convinced everyone that the best time to go to the dentist is *before* your teeth hurt—that routine dental care will help your teeth remain healthy for a long time. It is important to remember that, just like your teeth, your spine experiences normal wear and tear—you walk, drive, sit, lift, sleep, and bend. Regular chiropractic care can help you feel better, move with more freedom, and stay healthier throughout your lifetime. Although you can enjoy the benefits of chiropractic care even if you are only treated for a short time, the real benefits come into play when you make chiropractic care a part of your lifestyle.

Frequently Asked Questions

What is a chiropractic adjustment?

The chiropractic adjustment is a gentle controlled force applied to a particular vertebra, typically in the spine, intended to restore normal position and movement. Adjustments are important for restoring body alignment, balance, and reducing stress on the nervous system. Because of the fact that the nervous system is that master controller of all muscles and organs in the body, removing stress on the nervous system through chiropractic adjustments will frequently lead to improved health in the entire body.

How many adjustments will I need?

The total number of adjustments you need depends on five main factors: 1) your age, 2) your overall health, 3) the severity of your condition, 4) how long you have had your condition, and 5) what your ultimate goals are. If you are young, in good health, and have a mild condition that occurred very recently, you will need far fewer adjustments than if you are older, in poor general health, and have been struggling with a problem for many years. The total number of adjustments you will need also depends on whether you are just interested in reducing the pain you are currently experiencing, or are interested in creating optimal long-term health and wellness.

Will adjustments hurt?

No. The amount of pressure applied during an upper cervical adjustment is so minimal that my patients hardly feel much at all during the adjustment. Most people feel better very quickly, if not immediately after being adjusted.

Do I still need to see the chiropractor if my pain is gone?

It is very common for pain to disappear long before the total correction of your condition is attained. As in our earlier discussion, pain is not a very good indicator of health. Often times people are completely unaware of problems that are developing in them because there is no pain associated with them. Consider heart disease, cancer, diabetes—the three top killers—they don't have any symptoms at all until they have become very advanced. The same is true with cavities in your teeth—there is usually no pain until a cavity becomes severe. The point is that just because you are no longer experiencing pain does not mean that your problem no longer exists. It is important to continue being cared for so that the underlying cause of the pain can be corrected.

Routine chiropractic care is one of the simplest ways to maintain the health of your body. Numerous research studies have shown that people who receive regular chiropractic care suffer fewer illnesses, injuries, and degenerative diseases, and they report a better overall quality of life. In spite of the health benefits of chiropractic care, many people have never been to a chiropractor, most often because they don't really understand what chiropractic care is all about.

The bottom line is that chiropractic care is a safe, effective care for people suffering from a wide range of physical complaints, such as headaches, neck pain, low back pain, carpal tunnel syndrome, thoracic outlet syndrome, stomach and gastrointestinal complaints, wrist, elbow and shoulder pain, knee, hip and ankle pain, scoliosis, otitis media, and a host of other problems. While most of these disorders resolve within a few weeks or months, routine chiropractic care will help ensure optimal health for life.

Can Chiropractors prescribe medication?

Currently, chiropractors choose not to prescribe medications, although I may refer someone to another provider for prescription medication if I deem it necessary. However, in most cases, patients are better off with physical, rather than chemical, solutions for physical problems.

4

NUCCA Chiropractic

The field of chiropractic has always had in its foundation the adjustment of vertebrae to remove subluxations that interfere with normal central nervous system function. Chiropractic relies on manually adjusting the spine rather than on drugs or surgery, as with traditional medicine. What most people don't realize is that not all forms of chiropractic care are the same.

One form of chiropractic care is the method developed by the National Upper Cervical Chiropractic Association (NUCCA). Whereas typical chiropractic adjusts individual segments of the spine, the NUCCA method concentrates on aligning the entire spine through the top cervical vertebra. A specific focus on the upper cervical (neck) region is not new to the chiropractic field. It evolved during the 1920s from research conducted by Dr. B.J. Palmer at the Palmer Chiropractic Clinic in Davenport, Iowa.

Chiropractors have long focused on the top of the spine but not because they wanted to help headaches and neck pain. Due to the proximity of the top of the spinal cord to the brain (i.e., the brainstem), chiropractors who focus on this area of the spine have the greatest ability to influence the entire nervous system and human function. The brainstem is responsible for the function of nearly every body system. The higher in the spine that the adjustment is administered the more areas of the body that can be positively influenced.

Dr. Palmer discovered the upper cervical spine was a very common location for subluxations. He viewed subluxation as an interference with the innate intelligence or the body's natural healing ability. His system placed emphasis on alignment of the skull and the first and second vertebrae, which began the development and refinement of correcting upper cervical misalignments. He believed that if just the right amount of effort moved the vertebra in the right direction, it would stop on the center. This procedure did not involve the twisting and turning commonly associates with chiropractic. Instead, a quick flick of pressure is applied against the atlas vertebra to bring it back towards center.

In the late 1940s, Dr. Ralph Gregory, a graduate of Dr. Palmer's college, started working with Dr. John Grostic. Together, they studied the unique biomechanics of the upper cervical region to determine the different ways in which the vertebrae could shift from a normal position to a subluxated position. This involved very careful x-ray measurements of the joint surfaces and degrees of misalignment, and then applying mathematical formulas to plot exact directions to approach the misaligned vertebra and to reset them back toward their normal supporting functional position. An inherent quality to any force is direction, and more than ever before in the practice of chiropractic this element was being taken into account with a precise application. The more accuracy in determining the position of the misaligned vertebrae prior to care, the greater the probability of a more complete correction or reduced subluxation. Additionally, the accuracy of the upper cervical correction requires the least amount of force necessary to obtain the desired result. For example, one could kick a door open or one can get the key and open the door rather easily with minimal force, attaining the same result.

For the next fifteen years the two doctors developed and refined ways of measuring and distinguishing the unique features of the subluxation of the Atlas, or C1, so a documented and accurate correction could follow. From this partnership came the beginnings of a system of chiropractic that went beyond standardized adjusting involving a high force or strong depth. The initial post-graduate course for doctors who want to expand their expertise in adjusting the upper cervical area was called the Grostic technique.

In 1966, Dr. Gregory formed the National Upper Cervical Chiropractic Association (NUCCA). The NUCCA and its research organization, NUCCRA (National Upper Cervical Chiropractic Research Association) are dedicated to conducting upper cervical research for patients, doctors, and the chiropractic profession. The NUCCA board of university professors and chiropractors administer research for seminars, lectures, and articles. Since its inception, NUCCA has given chiropractic more biomechanical data regarding C1 subluxation, its effects, and treatment protocol than any other entity.

NUCCA research has given the profession more biomechanical data than probably any other area of chiropractic in the past twenty years concerning the subluxation, its effects on the spinal column and human body, and how to restore its misalignments to the vertical axis, and has shown acceptable and measurable proof of the benefits of the chiropractic adjustment on the human body.

The Path to Healing through NUCCA Chiropractic Care

In many ways, the approach to chiropractic care is the opposite of traditional medicine, for it focuses on prevention and wellness, rather than treatment; being proactive, rather than reactive; approaching health holistically, rather than specifically; and attaining a level of optimal health, not merely the absence of overt disease.

Trained NUCCA specialists understand that once the upper spine is in balance, the communication of information from the brain to the body is undisturbed and the nervous system is better able to function, which allows the body in its normal ability to restore and maintain optimal health. NUCCA technique involves movement of the spine generated by the doctor's hands in a very special way. All adjustments are made according to findings from highly accurate, laser-aligned, x-ray information. A gentle and controlled pressure is placed against the first vertebra with tremendous control to limit excessive depth and to maintain the proper direction. With such shallow movements, the patient hardly feels any force applied during correction. Often, patients feel no force at all but only the touch of the doctor's hands over the area of the vertebra, either on the right or left side of the neck. Following an adjustment, follow-up x-rays are taken to verify that the proper correction has been achieved.

Patients under this form of care who have been treated by other forms of chiropractic immediately recognize the difference between the two systems.

NUCCA Chiropractic Care Focuses on Avoiding Illness, Not Treating It

Although many people with various health challenges obtain great results through NUCCA care, the underlying premise of wellness care is that the focus of care should be directed away from treating disease and toward promoting good health. Another way of stating this is that wellness care concentrates on two areas: disease prevention and health promotion.

We can all think of our health on a sliding scale; the illness-wellness continuum. Illness is the extreme on one side and wellness is the extreme on the other side of the continuum. The obvious fact is that we are all on the continuum. The not so obvious fact is that we are all constantly moving either toward illness or toward wellness. Nothing living stays still, we are dynamic organisms. Each and every day the behaviors you choose or those you do not choose either move you towards illness or towards wellness. A balanced spine with minimal nerve interference will always move an individual toward wellness no matter where they are on the illness-wellness continuum. Minimal nerve interference is as essential to a healthy lifestyle as is regular exercise, great nutrition, ample rest, and a positive mindset.

NUCCA Chiropractic Care Is Proactive, Not Reactive

It is widely recognized that many of our health problems are caused by our behavior. If we can identify what behaviors are risky, we can educate our patients as to these risks and help them modify their behavior accordingly. Thus there are two parts to this enterprise: 1) identifying, usually through population studies, specific risk factors for certain diseases (smoking as a risk factor for lung cancer, for example, or high serum cholesterol as a risk factor for heat disease), and 2) empowering patients to choose more health-oriented behaviors for themselves and their families.

NUCCA Chiropractic Care Is Holistic, Rather Than Specific

Your body is not merely a group of organs that just happen to reside close to each other—your organs all function together. What happens in one area of the body affects all others. Because of this, it is necessary to take a holistic approach to improving your health. It is necessary to improve the health of the whole body in order to improve the health of a sick or damaged area. Traditional medicine takes a very specific approach where they try to just affect one particular area of the body, either through drug therapy or surgery.

Although the NUCCA adjustment is delivered at the top of the neck it influences the entire spine and body. The NUCCA doctor uses the top vertebra as a tool to access the person's nervous system. By influencing one of the body's greatest control centers, the brainstem, the NUCCA correction has the potential to positively impact any and all systems of the body.

NUCCA Chiropractic Care Focuses on
Attaining Optimal Health

The biggest difference between wellness care and disease care has to do with how health is defined. Traditional medicine views health as an absence of measurable disease, where wellness doctors view health as a state of optimal body function, where all of your body's systems are working properly in a coordinated way. As we stated earlier, health is a complete state of mental, physical, and social wellbeing and not merely the absence of disease and/or infirmity. Health is when 100 percent of the body parts are functioning at 100 percent, 100 percent of the time.

5

Our Patients Speak

When I decided to consider Dr. Larry Arbeitman for chiro-practic treatment, I had been experiencing neck and shoulder pain for about three years. I had tried conventional chiropractic treatment, heating pads, and deep tissue massage without success. I had to take Motrin almost every night in order to sleep. All of these things seemed to help temporarily, but within a day, the same problems would return.

I was unable to do simply house chores like vacuum, laundry, iron, or even talk on the phone without major discomfort. By the end of the day, I was irritable, tired and had little patience.

I started treatment in December and after only the first adjustment, I felt a HUGE difference. By the next visit, I had stopped taking Motrin and felt less irritable. After only a month, I was able to start working out and I now have more energy

*than I could imagine. This is a life-altering experience and I
am truly grateful. I had nothing to lose by trying this technique
and I have gained my life back. Thank you.*

- Jeannine W.

*For a year and a half, I've suffered with trigeminal
neuralgia. In that time, I've seen my MD, Neurologist, acupun-
turist, and have even been prescribed medications-all without
satisfactory results.*

*Dr. Gertner and his staff made me feel very comfortable
and after about three visits, I started noticing some relief. I've
been under care now for a couple of months and I'm now able
to eat, brush my teeth, and shower without pain. This was all
impossible before I started care at UCC. There have been some
other unexpected changes in other areas of my life as well.
I now have less back pain, feel more relaxed and have more
energy.*

*The only way I can describe how Upper Cervical Chiro-
practic has helped me is that it's "unbelievable." The is the only
treatment I would suggest to someone with trigeminal neuralgia.
Medical treatments and medications only helped manage my
symptoms. At UCC, they actually treated the cause.*

- Patricia G.

I have been an allergy sufferer for years. My allergies are year round and keep me from being able to enjoy the outdoors. After being on numerous inhalers and medications, allergy shots were the last option. So, I started receiving two allergy shots every other week. In spite of this, during the fall and spring, I could barely go outside or have the windows open.

I began treatment with Dr. Arbeitman in May, 2005 and have not found it necessary to have an allergy shot and have not suffered an allergy attack since then. I feel 100% better. I plan to continue treatment because the care I receive is training my body to be healthier and not rely on pills, shots, or inhalers to get through the day.

- Kylie

For the past 10 years I have suffered with very limited range of motion in my neck as well as tender sore spots all along my spine. I lost a lot of strength in my left hand and arm, and the pain in my right his was becoming so severe that I had to walk with a cane.

Before meeting Dr. Gertner, I had gone to three different neurologists and an acupuncturinst. I did not have any relief of my symptoms and became very frustrated.

Within the first two months of treatment with Dr. Gertner, the motion in my neck has improved dramatically, my spine is no longer sore and the pain in my hip is gone! I have regained strength in my left hand and arm, and I no longer have to

*walk with a cane. All of this with such a gentle, non-invasive
procedure. It's a miracle!*

- Florence S.

*Overall, I consider myself to be in pretty good health, but
I kept getting headaches every week, or so. Since I never knew
when they were going to hit, I kept a bottle of Tylenol in my
purse. Sometimes the Tylenol would help, other times, I just
had to sleep off the headache. As an elementary teacher, the
headaches affected my job because I could not give the students
my 100% attention.*

*Since beginning care with Dr. Arbeitman, I feel wonderful.
I haven't had a headache in months and I no longer have to
carry a bottle of Tylenol with me everywhere I go. Not only are
my headaches gone, but my energy level has been great and my
overall health feels like it has improved.*

- Nicole T.

*I have suffered with a burning sensation on the left side
of my back and a pinched nerve in my neck for the past two
months. The burning went from my back to my chest and under
my left arm and was so severe that it would almost bring me to
the point of crying.*

*Before seeing Dr. Gertner I saw a traditional chiropractor
and an orthopedic surgeon. The chiropractor adjusted me but*

it didn't help. The orthopedist took a bone scan and CAT scan, but found nothing.

My nephew was a patient of Dr. Gertner and recommended him to me. Although it was an 84-mile drive for me to Dr. Gertner's office, I was willing to give it a shot. I saw improvement in my condition within a day of the first procedure being performed, and after one month, I am 97% better.

I consider the procedure from Dr. Gertner a miracle. He is extremely conscientious. May God bless him and all who share in his work.

- Al M.

Initially I came to Upper Cervical Chiropractic due to what I was experiencing from a previous car accident and fall down a flight of stairs. The upper right hand side of my neck ached and I had recurring pain in my lower back. Traditional chiropractic, ibuprofen, and massage did not improve my overall health. Because of what I was experiencing I was not able to even pick up my youngest child. I also was unable to exercise at all.

After my upper cervical adjustments my health has improved considerably. I feel awesome! I am able to run everyday again. Even if I do feel tight, it gets better with just a little stretching or walking. I can carry my son again with ease! I will continue with my wellness care because I believe continuous care will keep my body in a great place and help my overall wellbeing.

Even the pain that I was experiencing from the injuries of ten years ago has improved with Dr. Larry's care. What would I tell others considering Upper Cervical Chiropractic care? Go, go, go and don't be afraid. It definitely is a different kind of chiropractic care. You will feel better after!

\- Jessica S.

I have suffered with low back pain for the past 20 years. After five unsuccessful back surgeries, I believed that I would be like this forever. I had been an avid mountain bike rider, but that lifestyle was just not an option for me anymore. I was referred to Dr. Gertner to discuss his finances. In conversation we discussed my situation, and with much skepticism, I decided to become a patient.

It is now hard to believe that such a gentle adjustment can have such amazing results. I do not know how to put into words the difference I feel. I sleep better, concentrate better, my balance is improved and I have no more pain. This is the best I've ever felt. Now that I am living without pain, I am able to enjoy the time I spend with my family much more. I can also coach lacrosse and am able to participate with the kids.

\- George R.

I was experiencing motor tics, constant, uncontrollable jerking of the head and neck. It seemed that I had tried every-

thing. I had been to physical therapy, tried muscle relaxers, and pain medication. I had been to a neurologist. I then made the decision to try botox injections to deaden the nerve. I was evaluated at a hospital for Parkinson's and Movement Disorders. This challenge was affecting many areas of my life. I had a problem driving and controlling the car. I had problems with balance - I walked into walls. I felt embarrassed when these situations occurred. At home all I wanted to do was lie down to support my head and stop the movements.

Now that I have been adjusted and been under care at Upper Cervical Chiropractic my uncontrollable movements are 95% eliminated. I know that continuing on wellness care is important so that I don't go back to where I was. I was so unhappy before. I would tell others considering care at Upper Cervical Chiropractic that this is different from traditional chiropractic care. There is no "cracking" or twisting of your head. I tell everyone who will listen that they should try it. They will see the difference for themselves. My wife was unsure about chiropractic care for 40 years - just seeing my improvement made her try it herself!

- Marty L.

For the past five years, I have suffered with neck pain, headaches, and numbness in my arms and hands. These symptoms were the result of an auto accident in 1999. I have seen my family doctor, an orthopedic surgeon, neurologist, and have been through pain management—all without success.

After only three visits with Dr. Gertner, my pain was reduced and I stopped taking my pain medication. The treatments are painless, and knowing that it is working makes every day better. I recommend Upper Cervical Chiropractic to anyone who suffers with chronic pain. It works and I am proof!

- Doug G.

A cervical spine injury had occurred many years ago. I had pain on the right side of my head and neck, shoulder stiffness, an inability to turn my head right and pain upon bending forward to look down. I tried many options; orthopaedics-Xrays, an MRI, physical therapy, a pain management doctor, did facet blocks, had epidural, radio frequency waves to deaden nerves, acupuncture, and naproxen. The chronic pain affected my home-life and relationships. It caused me to be stressed and annoyed. I stopped exercising because it made it worse. Cooking, cleaning and gardening were all painful leaning forward. My sleeping and sex life were affected. I did not want surgery so I decided to try Upper Cervical Chiropractic.

After my upper cervical adjustments I am so happy and relieved that things have improved, so much! I can turn my head right, and I can bend down with almost no pain. I resumed my gym workout and swimming. Sleep and sex are better. Dr. Larry insisted that I would heal-and I did! I know I will need continued care to feel good.

I still have the injury I've had for 18 years, but I know I need to keep in alignment to stay healthy. What would I tell others who are considering Upper Cervical Chiropractic care, but who are unsure about it? Be patient, trust Dr. Larry. Learn how not to aggravate your condition. Sometimes I had to use my hands to lift my head back up after bending forward and there were lots of crunching sounds. This has helped me to avoid surgery, improved my range of motion, and lessened the pain tremendously. It also allowed me to return to the activities I love like working out and swimming. I feel happy and hopeful and thankful to Dr. Larry. He has so much passion for his practice. I'm glad I hung in there with him.

- Lynn T.

A few months ago, my son fell out of a shopping cart and landed on his head. Since then, he has been wetting his bed every night.

I had been under the care of Dr. Gertner, myself, for only a few weeks, when I saw literature suggesting that children who wet their beds may get results through upper cervical chiropractic. Knowing how gentle and specific the adjustment was, I decided to have my son begin care.

We saw results immediately after the first visit. He no longer wet the bed. His is now more relaxed and alert at night,

---

he wakes up on his own to use the bathroom, and he now wakes up happier and proud of himself because he is a "big boy."

- Jah'Noah

As a young high school student, I found myself having a tight neck, headaches, constantly feeling fatigue, and body pains. My social life suffered, as well as my ability to play sports, and my school work became a burden because I was always tired. Since being evaluated by Dr. Larry, and becoming a practice member, I am able to go out everyday with my friends, play sports, and study more intently. Thanks to Dr. Larry I feel like a brand new person.

- Sarah G.

For the last year, I've suffered with relapsing and remitting multiple sclerosis. Some of the symptoms that I've been suffering with include tremors, poor circulation, neck and back pain, loss of coordination, fatigue, asthma, and insomnia. I've been to neurologists for this condition without satisfaction.

What I like most about Dr. Gertner's care is its effectiveness. It is simple, non-invasive, and without any side effects. Immediately after the first correction, I felt improved circulation in my legs and feet, less leg cramping, and I slept great for the first time in months.

I've been under care now for six months and UCC has helped me control my MS symptoms without medication. My tremors are almost gone and I am able to keep my hands steady. I now have much less spasticity, I sleep better, have less neck pain, better circulation, more energy, better concentration, and I no longer suffer from asthma!

- Don O.

Initially I had stiffness, numbness, poor mobility, leg discrepancy, pelvic subluxation, and a misaligned neck. I tried magnetic therapy for neck, traction, and physical therapy. The physical therapy gave me temporary relief for stenosis. My activities were limited. I couldn't do chores that I used to do. I had to use a cane when away from the house.

Now I have a return of mobility, my energy has increased, allowing me to become more active. Numbness has been replaced with circulation and feeling despite the pain which does not deter my ability to move. I plan on continuing with wellness care to resume doing regular activities and chores in addition to regular exercises such as bicycling and gardening in order to stay healthy without the use of a cane. Periodic check-ups should be in order.

I would tell others considering Upper Cervical Chiropractic care not to hesitate making an appointment if they want to improve their overall performance in whatever they do. If there are any questions one shouldn't be afraid to ask, if they want to be healthy!

- Leo A.

A virus, that had put me in the hospital, left me with extreme weakness, and pain. I was also dizzy, had blurry vision, headaches, tingling and confusion. This went on for five months. I saw specialists in neurology, infectious disease, rheumatology, and ophthalmology. I tried heating pads, pain killers and bed rest. Attendance at school was reduced to 3-4 hours a day and I stayed in bed the rest of the day. I couldn't work, do gymnastics, or go out with friends. At Upper Cervical Chiropractic of Monmouth, under Dr. Arbeitman's care, most of my symptoms disappeared. I noticed something happening within a week and felt healthier within 2 weeks. I am now back to school and gymnastics full-time. All the prior doctors and hospitals wanted to cover up my symptoms with drugs but Dr. Larry wanted to help my body heal. Give it a try you have nothing to lose and everything to gain.

- Stephanie L.

The migraines, headaches, and dizziness I was suffering from were crippling and debilitating my life. I no longer was able to run around and play with my children and wife. I felt that the best years of my life were over, and I am only 37. I have tried traditional chiropractic, pills, orthopedics, neurologists, physical therapy, and an ear, nose and throat doctor and received no relief. They told me that I have to deal with this pain for the rest of my life. I started to look around at other options. That is when I found Upper Cervical Chiropractic of Monmouth on the Internet headed by Dr. Larry Arbeitman and sent him an email. After the initial consultation, I knew Dr. Larry was special. His confidence, thoroughness, and compassion gave me a renewed feeling of hope. Dr. Arbeitman's concern is on his patients' recovery and well-being which is rare. The technique performed by Dr. Larry Arbeitman is the most amazing thing I ever experienced.

- Bob J.

I had been to two neurologists, an ENT doctor, tried antivert, had a CAT scan, and an MRI. I was not finding any help with the vertigo that I was experiencing. After seven weeks of conventional doctors, and trying to get appointments, then referrals. Nothing was actually done. My life was on hold. I couldn't work, and at times I couldn't read or watch TV. Being out in stores also bothered me. Then I found Dr. Larry Arbeitman at Upper Cervical Chiropractic and after beginning care began to see improvement. Now I am tremendously improved. I am back to work after 3 months. My first day back I was even able to do schoolwork that evening! After just 2 visits I felt much improved and after 8 visits, I was able to return to work. To maintain the proper alignment of my spine and continue on the path of good health I plan to continue with regular adjustments.

- Kathy L.

I was a migraine sufferer for many years, which limited my ability to work at times. I tried everything from over the counter medications to receiving prescriptions for my headaches and I could not find relief for my headaches. Through word of mouth I heard about Upper Cervical Chiropractic of Monmouth and made an appointment. I was a bit skeptical due to a previous experience I had. After meeting Dr. Arbeitman, he changed all my views about chiropractic with his gentle manipulation treatment and kind manner. Today, I have been headache free for about six weeks and even began running again. I highly recommend Dr. Arbeitman to anyone who wants relief!

- Ken T.

About Dr. Larry Arbeitman

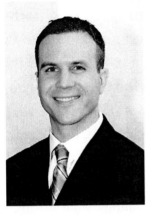 Dr. Larry Arbeitman is the founder of Upper Cervical Chiropractic of Monmouth (www.uccofmonmouth.com). He has dedicated his career to serving his community by empowering every man, woman and child to select upper cervical chiropractic care as a part of their wellness lifestyle. He is committed to being the premier Upper Cervical provider in the Northeast through public health education and technical excellence in the healing art of Upper Cervical Chiropractic.

Dr. Arbeitman graduated Magna Cum Laude, second in his class, from Logan College of Chiropractic in St. Louis, Missouri. He obtained his first Bachelor of Science degree in Kinesiological Sciences from the University of Maryland at College Park and a second Bachelor of Science degree from Logan College. The doctor is board certified in the state of New Jersey and by the National Board of Chiropractic Examiners. Throughout his educational career, he was a multiple scholarship recipient and accumulated several awards for academic achievement and exemplary clinical performance.

Dr. Arbeitman provides a vitalistic approach to patient care, which includes spinal and nervous system care, lifestyle management, work habit advice, fitness evaluations/programs and sound nutritional advice. He believes wholeheartedly that the relationship between the doctor and the patient is a key component to the healing process. He notes that the word "Doctor" means educator and that he serves as a patient's personal wellness coach.

Dr. Arbeitman has studied directly under some of the world's most renowned doctors and researchers in order to deliver the highest level of patient care. He has exceeded the normal Chiropractic educational requirements and has devoted hundreds of hours of extracurricular time at seminars and courses. Upper Cervical Care is extremely safe and Dr. Arbeitman has worked on professional athletes, newborns, pregnant mothers-to-be and seniors.

Dr. Arbeitman frequently lectures on various wellness topics for organizations, corporations and educational institutions. He has been a key note speaker at Farliegh Dickinson University, Logan College of Chiropractic, Quest Diagnostics, U.S. Coast Guard Junior Seamen and other venues. The doctor conducts and advanced seminar series in his office comprised of four workshops: Wellness 101, Eat Wellness, Move Wellness and Think Wellness.

Dr. Arbeitman has authored a dissertation on the effectiveness of chiropractic in the treatment of Sciatica and the Lumbar Disc Herniation.

The doctor holds active membership status with the National Upper Cervical Chiropractic Association (NUCCA), the Association of New Jersey Chiropractors and the Chiropractic Leadership Alliance.

About Dr. George Gertner

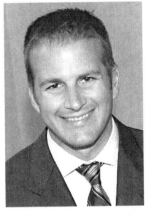

Dr .George Gertner is a family man, healer, philanthropist, mentor, public speaker, and founder of one of the world's busiest Upper Cervical Chiropractic clinics. Upper Cervical Chiropractic of New York, PC (www.ucc-ny.com), was established in 2002 and has quickly become the standard of excellence in the profession. Located in White Plains, it is less than 30 miles from New York City, and attracts patients from all over the world.

Dr. Gertner received his bachelors degree in biology from Hofstra University in Hempstead, New York before moving to Atlanta, Georgia to attend Life University. At the time Life was the largest and considered to be the most prestigious of all the chiropractic colleges.

Before graduation, Dr. Gertner had a severe injury to his lower back. For more than a year he was adjusted using every traditional chiropractic procedure available but still suffered with severe pain.

After almost giving up on a profession that Dr. Gertner spent the last 4 years dedicating his life to, he finally met a chiropractor who changed his life. The chiropractor specialized in an advanced spinal correction procedure developed by NUCCA (National Upper Cervical Chiropractic Association).

Immediately after the first visit, Dr. Gertner began to feel the amazing results of Upper Cervical Care. His body began to "heal itself" and the relentless pain that had plagued him now quickly left his body.

Dr. Gertner spent the next two years learning from one of the best Upper Cervical doctors, learning in the same office that helped change his life. After two years, Dr. Gertner returned home to New York to open his own office. He currently is one of only 5 NUCCA chiropractors in New York, and less than 300 worldwide.

Dr. Gertner has been featured numerous times in Chiropractic Monthly Magazine for his expertise in treating Trigeminal Neuralgia and Myofascial Pain. Dr .Gertner has lectured in local hospitals discussing the treatment of Trigeminal Neuralgia with Upper Cervical Chiropractic.

Since Upper Cervical Chiropractic helped him regain his life back, Dr. Gertner has found his Purpose. Through this specialty in chiropractic, Dr. Gertner has dedicated his life to helping those people who suffer hopelessly with chronic pain. It is his intent, that by reading this book, he is able to give you ... The Gift of Hope.

CPSIA information can be obtained at www.ICGtesting.com
Printed in the USA
BVOW030727240212

283723BV00006B/2/P

9 781933 889337